# SUPERFOODS
## FOR THE BRAIN

102 Nutrient Rich Foods To Strengthen
Your Mind & Improve Your Memory!

by Jennifer James

Published in Great Britain by:

LeadsClick
26 York Street
London
W1U 6PZ

© Copyright 2013 – Jennifer James

ISBN-13:978-1494430962
ISBN-10:1494430967

# Table of Contents

# INTRODUCTION:
# HOW TO EAT YOUR WAY TO OPTIMUM BRAIN HEALTH

What if you could improve your cognitive functioning, memory, focus, mental health and mood by changing the way you eat?

What if, by incorporating this special class of foods known as "superfoods" you could reverse the effects of aging and mental wear and tear to achieve greater brain health and potential?

No, superfoods aren't lab-created, artificially fortified, bionic substances designed by science to replace foods or help you reach your maximum mental and physical potential. It is so much simpler than that. These foods, rather, are the very best of what nature has to offer - the richest sources of vitamins, nutrients, anti-oxidants, phytonutrients, polyphenols, fiber and other health promoting elements.

# What are Superfoods?

Superfoods are the fruits, vegetables, natural fat sources, proteins, herbs and spices that boast a preponderance of health enhancing properties. They are recognized for their positive contribution to health and wellness.

While each superfood will have its own special properties and health offerings, most are known for being anti-inflammatory and high in antioxidants. They protect the body's vital organs and systems, repair damage, restore tissues and even lower risk of disease.

You may find, after studying this guide, that some of your favorite foods are superfoods!

# Why are Superfoods so Important?

In modern society our bodies are bombarded with free radicals and other pollutants that threaten our health and lead to premature aging, hormone disruption, weak immunity and even weight gain. But the effects aren't only on our bodies. Our brains also experience wear and tear. When we consume processed foods high in sugar, sodium, industrial fats and other chemicals, we sap our mind's ability to function. Have you ever noticed, for example, what a lunch of fried food does to your afternoon work performance? The belly is full and the brain is fuzzy. We combat it with a large cup of coffee or a candy bar to spike our blood sugar and hopefully give us the energy we lost on the unhealthy lunch.

What if it were possible to break that unhealthy cycle and experience focus, concentration and mental energy naturally? What if it were possible to leap the 3 o'clock slump and sail through the afternoon feeling productive, upbeat and energetic?

Many think they can pop a few vitamin supplements and then forget about what they eat. It isn't exactly that easy. Instead, we need to change the balance of our diet in favor of superfoods. These foods are nature's multivitamins, providing not only the nutrients that your body and brain needs, but also the satiation, great taste and increased vitality we all want out of the food we eat.

As you will see in the guide, one of the main benefits of superfoods is that they are highly nutrient dense. In short this means that with superfoods, you get the most bang for your buck - these foods really deliver! With superfoods, high levels of vitamins and nutrients are naturally packed into each bite. No empty calories, simple carbohydrates or unnecessary chemicals here; these foods are pure and unadulterated, as nature intended them. And because these foods so perfectly meet your body's nutritional needs, they are also abundantly satisfying and filling. While it's easy to eat an entire bag of nutrient depleted yet high calorie potato chips, superfoods fill you up. You'd be challenged to eat more than your really need.

# Superfoods and their Impact on the Brain

While the benefit of superfoods on the body is well documented and understood, it is the impact of superfoods on the brain that has become most intriguing in recent years. What positive effects can superfoods have on cognitive functioning, mental sharpness and even mental illness and mood?

Clean eating leads to clean, clear thinking. Superfoods provide the energy, vitamins, minerals, healthy fats and amino acids the brain needs to reach peak performance. Cognition, memory, retention and mental quickness are all improved in relation to an improved diet high in superfoods. Superfoods naturally help your brain work smarter.

And they protect the brain too. The lion's share of the battle against brain deterioration is combatting the free radicals that threaten the tissues of system of the body. This is the superfood's domain. Their antioxidant properties combat free radical damage in order to ensure that the brain and body are guarded against wear and tear and thus have the best possible opportunity to achieve top performance over the course of the life cycle.

Many superfoods also help to regulate cholesterol. While this is vital for heart health, proper cholesterol levels also help to lower risk of stroke. Other superfoods found in this guide help to prevent blood clots which can cause severe brain damage.

## How to Use This Guide

This guide will show you how to choose the superfoods that will allow you to achieve your best brain and body health.

Begin by reading through the 102 superfoods to learn which foods are classified as superfoods and to understand how they can contribute to achieving optimal brain health and mental functioning.

Each entry contains the name of the food as well as a description and the part of the food conveys the greatest benefit. In certain cases, such as with some fruits, more potent benefits for brain and bodily health can be obtained by consuming the skin or by choosing a particular variety over another.

This guide helps you to navigate those details so as to get the very most out of the foods you eat. Each description also contains a list of the main vitamins minerals, amino acids and antioxidant properties in each food and what conditions these components can help fight against or promote.

After learning about each of the superfoods, choose a few of the recipes to begin incorporating these foods naturally into your diet and getting the most you can out of your food.

You will soon notice you feel more focused and alert and maybe even happier as many of the superfoods found in this book also have natural mood-boosting properties. In addition to eating yourself healthy, you may also be able to eat yourself happy. Give your brain the best nature has to offer by making your diet a superfood diet.

Lets's begin ...

# FRUITS

## Acai

Acai berries are full of fiber, antioxidants, omega-3 fatty acids (oleic, palmitic and linoleic acid), proteins and phytonutrients. Various flavonoids found in acai have anti-allergic, anti-inflammatory, anti-cancer and anti-microbial properties. Acai can help reduce cholesterol, blood sugar, and metabolic syndrome risk factors in overweight people. Their high antioxidant quality helps combat oxidative stress and lessen the likelihood of many chronic illnesses.

## Apples

Apples have plenty of micronutrients including vitamin A, B1, B2, B6, C, biotin, folic acid, malic acid and pantothenic acid. Apple peels contain phytochemicals such as quercetin, epicatechin and procyanidin B2 which can help prevent many diseases. Â Apple peel also has a lot of usolic acid - in animal studies, this has been shown to increase skeletal muscle and brown fat but decrease white fat, obesity, glucose intolerance and fatty liver disease. Apples have fantastic antioxidant properties and can reduce the risk of colon, prostate and lung cancer.

## Apricots

Apricots are full of vitamin A, C, tryptophan, fiber and potassium. Consuming apricots helps protect us from heart disease and is good for our eye health. The high concentration of beta-carotene helps prevent LDL (bad fats) from oxidizing. There is a lot of lycopene in apricots, so eating them means oxidative stress in our bodies is reduced. Tryptophan is the precursor to serotonin and niacin - it will aid sleep and act as an antidepressant.

## Bananas

Bananas contains a lot of vitamin B6 and fiber, necessary for efficient metabolism and a healthy gut. They also contain quite a lot of vitamin B1, B2, B3, B5 and B9. High in vitamin C, manganese and potassium. Consuming bananas may reduce men's risk of developing colorectal cancer and women's risk of getting breast and renal cell carcinoma. The amino acid tyrosine is in bananas and this can affect the production of dopamine.

## Blackberries

Blackberries are particularly high in Vitamin C, K and manganese. Vitamin C protects vitamin E and helps the absorption of iron. Vitamin C is an effective free radical scavenger so it reduces oxidative stress. It is involved with the production of many hormones and the synthesis of collagen and carnitine. Carnitine is required for the transport of fats in the body as they are broken down.

## Cherries

Sweet red cherries have a lot of vitamin C. Sour cherries happen to have more vitamin C and a high vitamin A content. When the body is under stress or trauma it will produce 'reactive oxygen species' (free radicals). Too many free radicals can lead to many different diseases. Vitamin C is a powerful antioxidant that will reduce our risk of getting chronically ill.

## Coconut

Coconut contains a lot of fat and much of this is 'saturated fat' but according to research, the medium-chain fatty acids, which are plentiful in coconut, have not been shown to correlate with high cholesterol levels or cardiovascular disease. Coconut contains good levels of magnesium which is essential for the production of enzymes involved in many biosynthetic processes as well as energy metabolism. In addition, potassium and vitamin B2 important for the nervous system, muscle contraction and energy release.

## Cranberries

Cranberries are packed full of vitamin C, E and the mineral manganese. Vitamins C and E are brilliant free radical scavengers. Vitamin C assists with various enzymatic reactions and the absorption of iron. Vitamin E protects red blood cells from getting destroyed thereby improving oxygen delivery. Manganese is involved with blood clotting and it synthesizes connective tissue and bones. It helps with breakdown of carbohydrate and fat plus it optimizes the function of vitamin E.

## Figs

Figs contain so many nutrients in high concentration, such as vitamin B1, B2, B5, B6, K, the minerals calcium, iron, magnesium, manganese, phosphorous, potassium and zinc. There is little this superfood doesn't do for you! Manganese is particularly high. This mineral helps with the detoxification of free radicals, assists with blood clotting. It produces connective tissue, bones, sex hormones and synovial fluid. Manganese is involved with carbohydrate and fat metabolism and helps vitamin E to function correctly.

## Goji berries

These berries are packed with calcium, potassium, iron, zinc, selenium, vitamin B2 and C. They are also have many phytonutrients such as beta-carotene and zeaxanthin. Calcium helps cells to communicate and is the major mineral in bones and teeth. Potassium enables muscles to contracts and will normalise blood pressure. Iron is an important component of haemoglobin and the oxygen carrying capacity of red blood cells. Zinc and vitamin C help to boost the immune system. Selenium is a good scavenger of free radicals and vitamin B2 aids energy metabolism.

## Grapefruit

Grapefruit has plenty of vitamin C, a vital nutrient to help build connective tissue and boost immunity. Along with 'lycopene', vitamin C is a vital antioxidant that will pick up and destroy free radicals and therefore prevent the onset of various diseases like cancer. This fruit provides a good deal of fibre and will help to promote a healthily functioning gut.

## Grapes

Grapes contain polyphenols in their skin may help to prevent vascular damage and high blood pressure. They are also fantastic antioxidants.

Grapes have many nutrients - they are high in B vitamins but they may take more credit for their large quantity of vitamin K which is important for preventing osteoporosis.

## Green olives

Green olives are high in monounsaturated fat. These are good fats that are helpful for lowering LDL cholesterol (bad fats) so they can lower our risk of heart disease. Green olives have a lot of vitamin E. Vitamin E helps to 'scavenge' free radicals from lipid degradation therefore limiting cell damage and they protect red blood cells from hemolysis (destruction of red blood cells). The sodium in olives can assist in the regulation of blood pressure.

## Kiwifruit

Kiwifruits are particularly high in vitamin C. They are high in vitamin K too. Vitamin C are the perfect antioxidant. They help to reduce free radicals in the body, lessening the chance of many chronic diseases. Vitamin C protects vitamin E and is promotes iron absorption. Vitamin K is associated with bone mineralisation - it can help prevent osteoporosis.

## Lemons

Lemons have plenty of vitamin C which assists with many enzyme reactions in the body and is involved with hormone, collagen and carnitine production. Vitamin C is a powerful antioxidant that will decrease the amount of reactive oxygen species and help prevent unwanted chronic diseases.

## Limes

Limes do not have quite as much vitamin C as lemons. They do have some iron which is an essential component of haemoglobin and myoglobin. High levels of iron ensure that cells in the blood and muscles can effectively bind to oxygen. Iron also assists with the production of energy in aerobic metabolism.

# Nectarines

These fruits contain much vitamin C plus they have a reasonable amount of vitamin B3 and E. Vitamin C is responsible for the synthesis of collagen. It is a free radical scavenger so it can help to reduce cell damage. B3 is beneficial for tissue respiration. It helps raise HDL cholesterol (good fats) and lower LDL fats (bad fats) so it help keep atherosclerosis at bay. Vitamin is an antioxidant which prevents the destruction of red blood cells.

# Oranges

Oranges are famed for their vitamin C content. They also come stocked quite high with vitamin B1, B5 and B6. The antioxidant vitamin C is brilliant at picking up free radicals so they help to prevent cell damage and it can help boost the immune system. The B vitamins are heavily involved with metabolism and the production of energy.

# Papaya

Papaya fruit has many nutrients. They contain a particularly high amount of vitamin C and B9. Vitamin C is a strong antioxidant and will reduce the likelihood of cell damage. It is also plays an important role in many enzymatic reactions. B9 or 'folic acid' is responsible for synthesis and repair of DNA. It helps produce health red blood cells reducing our chances of anemia. There are many phytonutrients in papaya such as lycopene and polyphenols which also act as antioxidants and can prevent arteriosclerosis.

# Pears

Pears are a great sources of dietary fiber - eating pears will keep your digestive system healthy. They have lots of different nutrients but vitamin C and also vitamin K. Vitamin C is essential for the production of many hormones and the synthesis of collagen, a protein which makes up the fibrous connective tissues in our bodies. Vitamin K can prevent low bone density.

# Pineapple

Pineapple is particularly high in vitamin B1, B6, C and manganese. B1 and B6 are key vitamins in the production of energy. They are essential for fat and amino-acid (protein) metabolism and the breakdown of sugar. B6 is also responsible for synthesis of neurotransmitters (communicators of the nervous system), histamine (involved with immune response) and haemoglobin. Vitamin C and manganese help to prevent cell damage and produce connective tissue. Manganese also promotes fat and carbohydrate metabolism.

# Plums

There are a high variety of vitamins and minerals in plums. They are particularly high in vitamin C, K and contain ingredients such as dietary fiber that can help stimulate the digestive system. Vitamin C assists with iron absorption and protects vitamin E. Vitamin K is important for bone mineralisation and can prevent osteoporosis.

# Pomegranate

A fruit of high nutrient content, pomegranates are high in vitamin B1, B5, B6, B9, vitamin C, vitamin K and manganese. It is the B vitamin 'king' and so is essential to eat for an efficient metabolism and energy production. Vitamin C, K and manganese together will help generate connective tissue and bone density.

# Raisins

Raisins contain a lot of B vitamins, mainly B1, B2 and B6. They are also high in the minerals iron, manganese, phosphorous and potassium. Eating raisins helps us to metabolise glucose, amino acids and fatty acids. Both iron and B6 are responsible for haemoglobin synthesis. Manganese helps blood to clot and to detoxify free radicals. Phosphorous is a vital component of bones and DNA, energy substrates and cell membranes. Potassium helps muscle to contract and regulates our blood pressure.

# Raspberries

Raspberries are quite high in the B vitamins, especially B5. Besides other nutrients, they have plenty of vitamin C, E, K and manganese. Consuming raspberries is especially important for carbohydrate and fat metabolism and for the synthesis of Coenzyme A (helps to transport and oxidise fat). Vitamin C and E are skilled at removing free radicals therefore may prevent diseases such as cancer or heart disease. Vitamin K and manganese are essential for health bones.

# Strawberries

Strawberries are a great source of vitamin B9, C and manganese. They also contain plenty of antioxidant flavonoids such as fisetin. B9 is important for cell division and growth and it helps produce healthy red blood cells. Vitamin C prevents cell damage and boosts the immune system. Manganese is an effective free radical which is needed for fat and carbohydrate metabolism.

# Watermelon

Over 90% of watermelon is water so it is a fantastic hydrator. It has numerous nutrients the main ones being vitamin C and lycopene. Vitamin C helps to get rid of damaging free radicals and synthesizes collagen. It is though that consuming lycopene may reduce our risk of cancer, cardiovascular disease and macular degeneration.

# GRAINS

## Barley

Barley has many B vitamins such as B1, B3 and B6. It delivers plenty of minerals and has mostly iron, magnesium, phosphorous and zinc. B vitamins are important for the metabolism of fat, protein and carbohydrate and the synthesis or red blood cells. They also help to reduce the likelihood of atherosclerosis by increasing high density lipoproteins (HDL fats). The minerals in barley are involved with energy metabolism, bone formation and tissue growth.

## Black rice

Black rice contains around 9g of protein per 100g serving. It has unusual health properties. It is extremely rich in anthocyanins which are good antioxidants that can prevent heart disease. Iron is important for the formation of haemoglobin and enhances the ability of red blood cells to carry oxygen to our cells. Black rice is very fibrous and is a wonderful aid to digestion.

# Brown rice

Brown rice has plenty of B vitamins and is highest in B6 which means it is particularly good for optimizing the nervous system messengers (neurotransmitters) and increasing the amount of histamine and haemoglobin we produce. Brown rice has an incredibly high amount of manganese so eat this rice if you are looking to improve blood clotting and enhance your connective tissue and bone health. Other minerals that you also find in a very high quantity are magnesium and phosphorous.

# Chia seed

Chia seed contains omega-3 fatty acids which help to lower LDL cholesterol and prevent us from getting heart disease. It is a highly nutritious food containing particularly large quantities of vitamin B1, B3, calcium, iron, magnesium, manganese and phosphorous. These seeds will encourage a better metabolism, strengthen our bones, improve the formation of red blood cells and have an antioxidant effect.

# Millet

Millet is packed with manganese, tryptophan (which gets converted to B3), magnesium and phosphorous. Millet is an important food for the repair of tissues and bone and helps to form healthy cell membranes. Manganese acts as a cofactor for many enzymes involved in the metabolism of glucose and magnesium forms an essential component of genetical material as well as the principal energy substrate in the body, ATP. Tryptophan is an essential amino acid responsible for serotonin, important for the alleviation of depression.

# Oats

A fantastically healthy food, oats are especially high in vitamin B1 and B5. There are large quantities of minerals in oats: iron, magnesium, phosphorous, potassium and zinc but that which tops the list by a long way is manganese. Manganese is a co-factor for enzymes which detoxify the free radical superoxide and it promotes healthy tissue formation. B vitamins are important for a functioning metabolism and energy production.

## Quinoa

Quinoa does not quite have as much protein as beans but it is one of the most protein rich 'cereals' and is high in fiber too. It good portion of all nine essential amino-acids. It has plenty of vitamin B1, B2, B6 and B9 so will help in metabolism and energy production. Other minerals in high concentration are iron for healthy red blood cells, magnesium for metabolism, phosphorous for bone formation and zinc for tissue growth.

## Rye

Rye is very high in manganese and also has a good amount of fiber, tryptophan, phosphorous and magnesium. Rye will promote a healthy digestive system. Tryptophan is an amino acid that is a precursor to the production of serotonin (which is controls gut movement and appetite). Phosphorous is an important element that makes up bone, genetic material and cell membranes. Magnesium can manipulate genetic material and energy substrates such as ATP.

## Spelt

Spelt is high in vitamin B1, B3, iron, magnesium, phosphorous and zinc. It can encourage metabolism and the production of HDL cholesterol (good fats) for the prevention of atherosclerosis. Iron improves the oxygen carrying capacity of red blood cells and is involved with energy production. Eating spelt will also help our bones and tissues to be strong.

## Wheat berries

Wheat berries contain good sources of vitamin B1 and B3 which are vital for energy production and keeping LDL cholesterol low. They are high in magnesium, phosphorous, copper, manganese and selenium. They play an essential role in various enzyme reactions, bone formation, protein synthesis and our protection against free radicals.

# Wild rice

Wild rice is high in protein, particularly the amino acid lysine and it is packed full of fibre. Wild rice is highest in zinc and manganese which are important for tissue growth and hormone production. Lysine helps to stabilise collagen and elastin, important components of smooth muscle such as blood vessels.

# OILS

## Canola oil

Canola oil is low in saturated fat and high in omega-3 fatty acids, the main one being 'oleic acid'. It lowers LDL cholesterol (bad fats), reduces inflammation and possibly increases HDL cholesterol - this helps to prevent cardiovascular disease.

## Olive oil

Olive oil contains mainly 'oleic acid', a fatty acid responsible for the lowering of low density lipoprotein cholesterol which can have all sorts of beneficial effects such as lowering blood pressure and reduce our risk of heart disease. Olive oil is also full of vitamin E and K so it is an excellent source of antioxidant potential, it can protect our red blood cells and enhance bone mass density.

# PROTEIN

## Almonds

Almonds have large amounts of manganese, magnesium, tryptophan, copper, phosphorous, vitamin E and B2. Almonds help lower LDL cholesterol and reduce risk of heart disease. Magnesium promotes healthy blood vessels. Potassium helps the nervous system, muscle contraction, blood pressure and heart function.

## Anchovies

Anchovies like many oily fish, contain high levels of omega-3 fatty acids and a good dose of the immune booster, selenium. They are a wise addition in a diet as the good fats help to eradicate free radicals. It's best to stick to unsalted anchovies to limit sodium intake.

## Cashews

Most of the fats in cashews are 'good fats'. They

help to lower LDL cholesterol and prevent heart disease. Cashews are especially high in vitamin B5 and B6 so eating these nuts are essential for macronutrients metabolism as well as the production of nervous system messengers 'neurotransmitters'. The cashew nut is packed full of minerals: iron, magnesium, manganese, phosphorous, potassium and zinc. These minerals are key for red blood cell production, connective tissue and bone generation, muscle growth and contraction. Cashews are full of the antioxidants alkyl phenols.

## Chicken

Chicken is a very lean sources of protein, the building block of all tissues in the human body. Chicken has good levels of vitamin A, B5 and iron. These minerals are essential for efficient growth and development, a healthy immune system, metabolism and red blood cell function.

## Chickpeas

Chickpeas are particularly high in the B vitamins,

B1, B6 and B9 so they are fantastic to eat for a well functioning metabolism. There is quite a lot of phosphorous and zinc. Phosphorous is an important element of DNA and cell membrane. Zinc aids the growth and development of tissues. Chickpeas have a very high B9 and iron content so they are helpful for preventing anemia.

## Eggs

Eggs provide all the essential amino acids needed for our diet. They are full of many nutrients such as vitamin A, B2, B5, B9, B12, Choline, vitamin D, phosphorous and zinc. They are good for eye health and energy production. Choline is normally classed as a B vitamin and is an important constituent of cell membranes. Vitamin D will help absorb calcium and is essential for bone density. Phosphorous forms our genetic material, DNA and zinc is responsible for the growth of muscle.

## Flaxseed

Flaxseed is very high in fiber and will promote a healthy gut. They have an amazingly high vitamin B1 and magnesium content. Flax is also a good source of other B vitamins, calcium, iron, phosphorous, potassium and zinc. Flaxseed has an impressive 19g of protein in each 100g. It helps our metabolism run smoothly, builds bone, cells and muscle tissue. The potassium helps transmit nerve impulses for muscle contraction.

## Hemp seeds

Hemp seeds contain plenty of essential fatty acids, specifically ALA and GLA (the good fats). These fatty acids can reduce inflammation in the body, are associated with a lower likelihood of heart disease and can prevent cancer. They are also beneficial for the nervous system, for example brain function and as for stimulating the gut.

# Kidney beans

These beans contains lots of vitamin B5 and B9, essential for carbohydrate and fat metabolism as well as cell division and healthy blood cells. Kidney beans also provide calcium, iron, magnesium, potassium and zinc - ideal for bone health, efficient metabolism, a normal blood pressure and tissue growth. Kidney beans are very high in protein and fiber, beneficial for tissue repair and a normal digestive system.

# Lentils

Lentils are densely nutritious. They are especially high in vitamin B1, B5, B6 and B9 (B9 is the most abundant). Lentils contains all the important mineral but are highest in phosphorous which essential for cell membrane, bone and genetic material formation. The B vitamins are crucial for energy metabolism but the high B9 produces healthy red blood cells and prevents anaemia.

# Peanuts

Peanuts high in protein and are filled with energy. They have been found to contain a very high concentration of free radicals which help to reduce the chance of heart disease and prevent cell damage, lessening our chances of getting cancer. Peanuts are very high in many B vitamins as well as magnesium, phosphorous and zinc. Important for a healthy metabolism, cell membrane formation and tissue development.

# Pinto beans

Pinto beans are particularly high in vitamin B12, molybdenum and fibre. Vitamin B12 is important in the synthesis of proteins. Molybdenum is responsible for the formation of many vital enzymes and waste disposal from the kidneys. Fibre can enhance the absorption of nutrients through the gut wall and has been shown to reduce the likelihood of bowel cancer.

# Pumpkin seeds

Pumpkin seeds are really high in protein, containing around 30g per 100g of seed. They supply us with many nutrients and are very high in vitamin B3, iron, magnesium, manganese, phosphorous and copper. B3 is essential for efficient glucose metabolism and it helps to raise 'good fats'. Iron improves our red blood cells ability to carry oxygen and is important for the prevention of anaemia. Magnesium, manganese and phosphorous play a role in metabolism, and the formation of bones and connective tissue. Copper offers protection against free radicals and assists with iron metabolism.

# Salmon

Salmon is a great source of protein which tops us our levels of vitamin D, B12, B3, tryptophan, selenium and phosphorous. This fish is high in omega-3 fatty acids - these reduce LDL cholesterol and maintain our arterial health. Salmon also contains amazing joint supporting peptides which research shows, improves insulin action and reduces inflammation in the gut. Vitamin D helps absorb calcium and along with phosphorous is essential for bone formation. B12 is needed for protein synthesis. Tryptophan is an amino acid which is thought to counteract the effects of depression and selenium is a good antioxidant.

## Sardines

Sardines are a great source of heart healthy omega-3 fatty acids. They have plenty of vitamin B12, D and B3, effective compounds for energy metabolism, calcium absorption and protein synthesis. Eat sardines to top up with tryptophan and sleep better, selenium for protection against free radicals and phosphorous to keep cell membranes strong.

## Sesame seeds

Sesame seeds are rich in protein. They have lots of iron, magnesium, phosphorous and zinc. They are important to eat for healthy red blood cells, a properly functioning metabolism, good bones and tissues. The high number of omega-3 fatty acids in sesame oil can protect us from cardiovascular disease.

## Sunflower seeds

Sunflower seeds are very high in vitamin B1, B6 and E. They contain lots of minerals such as magnesium, manganese and phosphorous. B vitamins are vital for energy production and vitamin E helps to protect red blood cells and scavenge harmful free radicals. Other minerals in sunflower seeds play an important part in energy production and healthy formation of bones and tissues.

## Tahini

Tahini provides a good quantity of B1, copper, manganese, phosphorous and the amino acid methionine. When compared to peanut butter, tahini has more fiber, less sugar and fewer saturated fats. Omega-3 fatty acids are 'essential' because our body can't manufacture them by itself. Tahini contains plenty of these 'essential fats' and will help lower our chances of getting cardiovascular disease - along with methionine they are important for the prevention of atherosclerosis (build up of fats on our artery walls). Tahini consumption is important for effective sugar and amino acid metabolism and it is loaded with antioxidant benefits.

## Tempeh

Tempeh is full of protein, fibre, vitamins and minerals. If you want a good top up of vitamin B2, manganese, copper, phosphorous and magnesium, tempeh is the food for you. B2 ensures that energy metabolism in the cell mitochondria is functioning well. Manganese and copper help reduce cell damage by diminishing free radical activity. Phosphorous is an important component of bone and magnesium forms part of our genetic material as well as the energy substrate, ATP.

## Tofu

It is now known that the antioxidant effects of tofu is related to the 'fermentation time'. If tofu is fermented for longer, then this can greatly increase its ability to eliminate free radicals. Tofu is particularly high in tryptophan, calcium, manganese and iron. Tryptophan can help regulate our appetite and improve our mood. Calcium and manganese are important for bone health and iron is an essential component of metabolism and red blood cells.

## Tuna

Eat fresh tuna for a satisfying dose of protein and omega-3 fatty acids. Protein helps in the generation of healthy tissue and good fats reduce our risk of atherosclerosis and heart disease. This fish is particularly high in vitamin D and phosphorous so it is very important for bone generation and the prevention of osteoporosis.

## Turkey

Turkey is a lean, white meat which provides an excellent source of protein, vitamin B3, B6 and phosphorous. It is important to consume for an optimum metabolism and healthy bones. Eating turkey can help prevent a build up of fatty plaque on our arteries, and the phosphorous in it will build strong cell membranes.

## Walnuts

Walnuts are rich in omega-3 fatty acids which are vital for the prevention of heart disease. They are especially high in vitamins B1, B6 and B9 which are important for energy production and red blood cell synthesis. For a good source of magnesium, manganese and phosphorous, make sure to eat walnuts as they will improve metabolism and bone density. Walnuts provide vitamin E as 'gamma-tocopherol' which is particularly beneficial in the fight against heart disease.

# HERBS AND SPICES

## Basil

Fresh basil has many nutrients. In particular, basil contains an extremely high amount of vitamin K so if you suffer from low bone density, basil should be of top priority in the diet. It is also very high in vitamin A and beta-carotene, important substances for optimum eye sight. There is quite a lot of vitamin C, iron and manganese in basil. These are beneficial nutrients for protection from free radicals, healthy red blood cells and a good metabolism.

## Chilli

Chillis are known for their vitamin C content and they have pretty good sources of many B vitamins and minerals but are especially high in vitamin B6. Vitamin C can help the absorption of iron in our diet and increase collagen (connective tissue) formation. Vitamin B6 synthesizes neurotransmitters (chemical signals in our nervous system) and is particularly important for the metabolism of proteins.

## Cinnamon

The spice cinnamon can replace refined sugar in our diets to help sweeten food. It is also high in the mineral manganese which is essential for the biological activity of many enzymes involved with free radical elimination. It helps with blood clotting and leads to the formation of sex hormones and joint synovial fluid.

## Coriander

Coriander has plenty of beta-carotene and vitamin A. It is a fantastic source of vitamin K and a good source of vitamin C and manganese. Vitamin A and C helps promote good eye health and optimum immunity. Manganese is an excellent antioxidant too and will encourage robust bone and connective tissue development.

## Himalayan sea salt

Salt is essential for life processes. Himalayan salt can help to regulate blood pressure, prevent muscle cramps during exercise, enhance bone strength and help with cellular pH balance in our cells. The salt is made up of huge number of different minerals. The pink colour in Himalayan salt is attributed to iron oxides which can strengthen the blood to help fight off disease.

## Mint

Mint can improve our digestion. It is high in vitamin A, C and manganese therefore it is packed full of antioxidants, which will attack disease forming free radicals. It helps with our metabolism and will promote the formation of healthy connective tissue and bones.

## Parsley

Parsley is packed full of vitamin A and beta-carotene therefore it has will help our eye health and act as an effective antioxidant. It is has lutein and zeaxanthin which reduce risk of AMD (age-macular degeneration). If you suffer from low bone density or osteoporosis, eat lots of parsley at it contains an almost unbelievable quantity of vitamin K. Parsley is also a good source of iron and vitamin B9 for healthy red blood cells as well as vitamin C for a boosted immunity.

## Paprika

Paprika is a dried powder derived from chillis. It is especially high in vitamin C. Vitamin C is a good free radical scavenger. It manufactures hormones, the amino acid carnitine and connective issue. It contains the phytochemicals xanthophyll, carotenoid and zeaxanthin.

# Vegetables / Salads

## Asparagus

Asparagus is made up of many B vitamins. It is a particularly good source of vitamins B1, B2 and K. These B vitamins are important for energy metabolism and vitamin K is good to eat to maintain optimum bone density.

## Avocados

Carotenoids give avocados their antioxidant properties - beta-carotene, alpha-carotene and lutein are the main ones. Avocados are high in phytosterols. These support our immune system. There are also many polyhydroxylated fatty alcohols in these fruits which are anti-inflammatory. Avocados contain plenty of fiber, vitamin K, folate, vitamin C, vitamin B5, potassium and vitamin B6 (B vitamins reduce homocysteine which promotes heart health).

## Beetroot

Betacyanin is a disease fighting phytonutrient that is plentiful in beetroot. Beetroot contains vitamin B9 which provides defense against colon cancer and birth defects. There is a lot of beta-carotene and fiber in beetroot which is recommended for good vision and a healthy digestive system.

## Bell peppers

Bell peppers are full of vitamin C and contain lycopene. Both ingredients are powerful antioxidant. They help to get rid of the disease inflicting free radicals. Vitamin C will give our immunity a big boost, it plays an important role in enzyme reactions during glucose metabolism and enhances our absorption of iron.

## Broccoli

Broccoli supplies us with a good dose of dietary fibre and therefore improves our digestive flow. It is a highly nutritious vegetable but is particularly high in vitamins C and K. Vitamin C is an antioxidant that will fight off free radicals and reduce our chances of getting heart disease or cancer. Vitamin C also helps us absorb iron and it generates connective tissue. Vitamin K is extremely important for building bone.

## Brussel sprouts

Brussels contain vitamin A as well as beta-carotene, lutein and zeaxanthin which are all powerful antioxidants and important for good eye sight. Eat your brussel sprouts for your daily dose of vitamins C and K. Vitamin C protects our cells from damage and helps to synthesize collagen. Vitamin K prevents osteoporosis.

## Carrots

Carrots are full of vitamin A which is excellent for our tissue growth and vision. The orange colour in carrots comes from beta-carotene. Along with lutein and zeaxanthin, these phytochemicals help to prevent age-related macular degeneration and having plenty of these in your diet will mean a better immune system and a lower chance of suffering from a chronic illness.

## Collard greens

Collard greens are highly dense in nutrients. They contain a lot of vitamin A and the carotenoids, beta-carotene, lutein and zeaxanthin. These provide antioxidant protection and a reduced likelihood of age-related macular degeneration (they protect the eyes). These greens are high in vitamin C, another good free radical scavenger and have many anti-cancer ingredients. They contain plenty of manganese and vitamin K to keep bones strong.

## Cucumbers

Cucumbers contain over 90% water so they can help to keep us hydrated. They have a good range of nutrients and are highest in Vitamin K which plays an important role in bone mineralization. They are a clever supplement to a diet belonging to anyone wanting to lose weight because of their low calorie content.

# Garlic

Garlic has numerous health benefits. It contains a huge amount of vitamins B6 and C plus good levels of the minerals calcium, iron, manganese, phosphorous and zinc. By consuming garlic, it is thought that we are protected to an extent against atherosclerosis, too much bad cholesterol and high blood pressure. Vitamin C is an antioxidant which prevents cell damage and helps protect us against cancer. Vitamin B6 is essential for protein metabolism. Selenium is also present in garlic and long with manganese defends us against free radicals.

# Ginger

Ginger root is made up of many B vitamins. It is especially high in B3 and B9 and therefore helps reduce our vulnerability to atherosclerosis and promotes very healthy red blood cells. If you are in need of free radical detoxification and healthy connective tissue, eat ginger because it has an incredibly large amount of manganese. Iron is also very high up on the list, a very important element for haemoglobin formation and the electron transport pathway in aerobic metabolism.

## Green beans

Green beans a very good source of most disease fighting vitamins and minerals. It is highest in vitamins C and K. Green beans contain the phytochemical 'miquelianin', an antioxidant that will help to get rid of the free radicals which are produced after exercise or at times of stress. Vitamin C boosts our immunity and vitamin K builds strong bones.

## Green cabbage

Cabbage contains a good range of vitamins and minerals with a wide array of health benefits. It is particularly high in vitamins C and K. By eating cabbage, our immune system and bone health will be improved. The antioxidant activity helps to reduce inflammation and protect our cells from free radical damage.

# Kale

Kale is a very popular superfood which is packed full of nutrient goodness. There is lots of vitamin A, C, K and carotenoids in kale and also plenty of manganese. Vitamin A is good for eye sight plus vitamin C encourages iron absorption and fights disease. Kale is extremely beneficial if we want to build bone density. Carotenoids and manganese are important for protection from free radical damage.

# Mushrooms

When mushrooms absorb sunlight, they then contain a good amount of vitamin D which is vital for bone health. Mushrooms are low in calories but provide nutrients such as vitamin B2, B3, selenium and potassium. Eating mushrooms means that we benefit from antioxidant protection and a healthy blood pressure.

# Mustard greens

Mustard greens contains high levels of vitamins A, B9, C and K as well as minerals such as manganese.

Vitamin A plays a role in enhancing our immunity and B9 helps prevent anaemia. Vitamin C is a free radical scavenger and will prevent the likelihood of diseases such as cancer. Vitamin K and manganese are great for bone density.

## Onions

Onions have many nutrients, the mains ones being vitamins C and B6. These compounds are important for iron absorption and haemoglobin function. Vitamin C is great for the immune system and helps to protect us from disease. B6 assists the metabolism of amino acids and lipids. In addition it helps to release glucose and provides with much needed energy.

## Peas

Peas are a healthy source of vitamin A, vitamin C and the carotenoids beta-carotene, lutein and zeaxanthin. All these are important for a healthy immunity and keeping free radicals to a minimum. Eat peas also for a good dose of vitamin K, iron, manganese, phosphorous and zinc.

# Pumpkin

Pumpkin's orange colour comes from the antioxidant carotenoid, beta-carotene. Pumpkin also contains the eye health boosting vitamin A, lutein and zeaxanthin. Pumpkin provides many of the B vitamins which are important for energy production and contains a lot of immune building vitamin C.

# Radish

Radish is a highly alkaline food, rich in the B vitamins but especially vitamin C and potassium. Radishes help our metabolism to function correctly and the antioxidant vitamin C protects vitamin E. Potassium is essential for optimum nerve signaling and muscle contraction.

# Red cabbage

Red cabbage contains a substance called sulforaphane which could increase enzymes that reduce the likelihood of various cancers. It is particularly high in vitamins C and K. So, we should eat red cabbage to increase our immunity, optimize the absorption of iron and strengthen our bones. The pigment in red cabbage originates from 'anthocyanins' which are chemicals that can inhibit growth of tumours.

## Rocket

This flavoursome herb has so many wonderful nutrients. Rocket provides a lot of vitamin A and it's precursor beta-carotene, both important for good eye health. There is a lot of anti-carcinogenic phytonutrients in rocket. This salad leaf contains plenty of vitamin K, necessary for blood clotting and strong bones, calcium for cell signalling, and potassium for maintaining a normal blood pressure.

## Romaine lettuce

Romaine lettuce is packed full of antioxidants such as vitamin C. It is especially high in vitamin A and B9, essential nutrients for eye health and well formed red blood cells. The dark pigment, chlorophyll has been shown to possess cancer-fighting properties.

## Red chard

Eat red chard to improve your eye health with its high vitamin and beta-carotene content. Chard is nutrient rich but in highest supply is vitamin C and blood clotting vitamin K. Chard provides antioxidant defense to prevent disease and optimum bone health.

## Spinach

Spinach is packed full of vitamin A and the carotenoids beta-carotene, lutein and zeaxanthin. These are important antioxidants that boost immunity and prevent eye damage. Spinach is particularly high in vitamins B9, C, K and highest in the mineral manganese. It is an essential vegetable to eat for healthy red blood cells, a good immunity and strong bones.

# Squash

Squash is very fibrous and healthy for our digestive system. It has much of the vitamin C and B6 we need, so is important for connective tissue formation and an efficient metabolism. It contains most of the B vitamins and therefore helps to release energy from the body's carbohydrate stores.

# Sweet potatoes

Sweet potatoes are packed full of beta-carotene which are thought to lower our chances of getting breast cancer and vitamin A, an important vitamin for tissue growth and immunity. High in vitamins B5, B6 and the mineral manganese, sweet potatoes are good for metabolism and getting rid of free radicals.

# Turmeric

Turmeric is a popular plant for the prevention of many diseases such as cancer and Alzheimer's. 'Curcumin' is a chemical in turmeric which also has anti-inflammatory, antibacterial, antiviral and antioxidant activities.

# OTHER SOURCES

## Agave

Agave has a lower glycemic index that sucrose
(table sugar) which helps to prevent glucose spikes,
the overproduction of insulin and type 2 diabetes.
Nevertheless, it is tastes sweeter than sugar and we
should choose 'raw' agave at it is manufactured at
lower temperatures which helps to protect the
beneficial enzymes.

## Cocoa

Cocoa 'solids' or 'powder' are the low fat part of
chocolate. This superfood is densely packed full of
minerals, especially iron, magnesium, manganese,
phosphorous and zinc. Cocoa is well known for its
high 'flavonoid' content. Scientific researchers have
shown that flavonols are linked to a lesser
incidence of heart disease and stroke.

# Green tea

Green tea has a really high concentration of flavonoids which powerful antioxidants and can help prevent certain types of cancer. There is ongoing research that suggests that green tea can lower cholesterol and may help reduce our percentage body fat.

# Milk

Milk is high in quality protein, which helps to rebuild muscle tissue. It has plenty of calcium, an essential nutrient for strong bones and teeth. It is especially high in vitamins B2 and B12 which play an important role in our metabolism and the synthesis or proteins. Plant milk is a healthy alternative to dairy and contains a good variety of necessary nutrients.

# Yoghurt

This calcium rich food is prepared using a mixed culture of 'good bacteria' that are essential to digestion. They help to stimulate cell growth but decrease the production of harmful bacteria. These bacteria can enhance our levels of vitamin B12 and provide defense against a whole host of diseases. Yoghurt is also rich in vitamins B2 and B6 so it is important to eat for energy release and proper haemoglobin function.

# SUPERFOOD RECIPES: WEEKLY PLANNER

## Monday: Breakfast

<u>Kick-start porridge</u>

### Ingredients:

- 2 cups oats
- 3 cups 2% milk
- 1 tsp cacao nibs
- 1/2 tsp cinnamon

### Directions:

Pour the porridge oats into a pan with the milk and simmer for 10 minutes. Let the porridge cool slightly. Sprinkle the cacao nibs and cinnamon on top of the porridge.

# Monday: Lunch

<u>Quinoa, broccoli and cashew salad</u>

**Ingredients:**

- 300g quinoa
- 200g tenderstem broccoli, roughly chopped
- 1/2 cup blanched cashew nuts
- 1 handful pumpkin seeds
- 1 handful mint leaves, finely chopped
- 1 handful parsley, finely chopped
- 4 cherry tomatoes, halved
- 4 scallions spring onion, finely chopped
- 2 tbsp olive oil
- 2 tbsp lemon juice
- 1 pinch Himalayan salt

**Directions:**

Cook the quinoa and then leave it to cool. Steam the broccoli until slightly cooked but with a 'crunch'. Heat some oil in a frying pan to lightly fry the pumpkin seeds and spring onions. Wait for the ingredients to cool and add them to the quinoa and broccoli. Mix in the cashews, herbs and tomato. Mix the olive oil and lemon juice together and pour over the salad. Add a pinch of salt to season.

# Monday: Dinner

<u>Cabbage salad with chilli tuna and black rice</u>

## Ingredients:

- 1/2 cup black rice
- 1 tsp olive oil
- 4 oz tuna fillet
- 2 red chillies, finely chopped
- 2 tbsp lemon juice
- Himalayan salt

*Cabbage salad*

- 1 carrot, roughly shredded
- 2 scallions spring onion, chopped into thin strips
- 4 oz red cabbage, finely chopped
- 4 oz red pepper, chopped into thin strips
- 1.5 oz cucumber, grated into thin strips
- 1/2 cup basil leaves, finely chopped
- 1 tbsp lemon juice
- 1 tbsp olive oil
- 1 clove garlic, crushed

## Directions:

Add the water to the black rice and heat until boiling, place the lid on the pan and lower the heat to simmer until the rice is cooked. For the cabbage salad, lightly fry the spring onions and red cabbage until slightly crisp. Mix up the carrot, red pepper, cucumber, basil, spring onion and red cabbage. Stir the lemon juice with the olive oil and garlic well to make a dressing. Pour the dressing onto the salad. Season the tuna with the salt, chillies and lemon juice. Heat the olive oil in a pan. Place the seasoned tuna onto the pan and lightly cook each side. Finish frying the tuna until it is just about cooked all the way through. Serve the fish with the rice and salad.

# Tuesday: Breakfast

<u>Bircher muesli</u>

- 200g rolled oats
- 400ml milk
- 1 apple (with skin)
- 1 tbsp agave syrup
- 150ml natural yoghurt
- Handful blueberries and raspberries
- Handful almond flakes

## Directions

Put the oats in a bowl to soak with the milk. Place them in the fridge for about an hour. Roughly grate the apple over the oats and mix in the honey and yoghurt. If the mixture is too thick, add a touch more milk or water. Lightly toast the almond flakes in a frying pan. Sprinkle the almond flakes and blueberries over the top of the oats.

# Tuesday: Lunch

<u>Chickpea and bean soup with a pumpkin seed and garlic topping</u>

## Ingredients:

- 6 cloves garlic, peeled
- 2 tbsp olive oil
- 15 oz red kidney beans
- 15 oz chickpeas
- 1lb vine tomatoes, chopped
- 3 cups vegetable stock
- 1 tbsp lemon juice
- Himalayan sea salt

*Pumpkin seed and garlic topping:*

- 1/2 cup pumpkin seeds
- 2 handfuls basil leaves
- 1 handful mint leaves
- 1 clove garlic (crushed)
- 1 tbsp lemon juice
- 2 tbsp olive oil

## Directions:

Pre-heat the oven to 400 degrees fahrenheit. Place the garlic cloves in pan and roast for 10-15 minutes. Add the tomatoes and roast for another

10-15 minutes or until the cloves are slightly browned and the tomatoes are soft. Place the garlic, tomatoes, beans and chickpeas into a blender and blend until smooth. Pour this mixture into a pan and heat until warm. Add in the lemon with the himalayan salt and pepper to taste. For the topping, finely grind the pumpkin seeds in a food processor. Mix in the basil, mint, crushed garlic, lemon juice and salt, then blend this. As the blender is still processing on low speed, add the oil until a thick sauce is created. Put a dollop of this sauce on the soup to serve.

# Tuesday: Dinner

Salmon, pinto bean and rocket salad.

## Ingredients:

- 4 oz salmon fillet
- 2 cloves garlic, crushed,
- 2 tbsp lime juice,
- 2 tbsp coriander, finely chopped
- 2.5 oz pinto beans
- 1 small red onion, finely chopped
- 1 tsp hemp seeds
- 1 tbsp olive oil
- 1 oz rocket
- 3.5 oz peas

## Directions:

Pre-heat the oven to 200 degrees Celsius. Mix together the crushed garlic, lime juice and coriander and marinate the salmon with these ingredients for 15 minutes. Cover and seal the salmon with foil and cook in the oven for 15 minutes. Rinse the beans and bring then to the boil with some water, and then simmer until cooked. In the meantime, simmer the peas until lightly cooked. Fry the onions with the hemp seeds until the onions start to brown and then remove from the heat. Add the cooked beans to the onions and seeds. Then stir in olive oil, rocket and peas. Serve the salmon fillet on top of the salad.

# Wednesday: Breakfast

<u>Wake-up smoothie with yoghurt and figs</u>

## Ingredients:

- 1.5 cups greek yoghurt
- 8 oz fresh figs, halved
- 1/2 cup sunflower seeds
- 1 tbsp agave syrup
- 1 pinch ground cinnamon

*Smoothie*

- 1 banana,
- 1 cup almond milk
- 1 handful frozen cherries
- 1 tbsp acai powder

## Directions:

Heat the sunflower seeds until slightly browned. Caramelize the figs in the agave syrup on a low heat in a pan. Put the figs and seeds over the yoghurt and dust the cinnamon across the top. To make the smoothie, add all the smoothie ingredients to a blender and process until smooth. Serve with a straw.

# Wednesday: Lunch

Spicy Turkey with pumpkin

## Ingredients:

- 1 tbsp olive oil
- 1 small red onion, chopped
- 1/2 green bell pepper, chopped
- 1/2 yellow bell pepper, chopped
- 1 clove garlic crushed
- 4 oz turkey mince
- 1/2 cup vine tomatoes, chopped
- 1 cup pumpkin puree
- 1 tsp paprika
- 1 pinch himalayan salt
- 1 tbsp greek yoghurt
- Parsley

## Directions:

Saute the onion in the oil over a medium heat. Add the green pepper, yellow pepper and garlic - cook until softened. Then add the turkey meat and cook through. Drain any excess water away. Then mix in the tomatoes and pumpkin puree. Sprinkle with paprika and salt. Lower the heat until just simmering for around 20 minutes. Place a small amount of greek yoghurt on the top with a parsley garnish.

# Wednesday: Dinner

<u>Chicken, mushroom and cashew stir-fry</u>

## Ingredients:

- 1/2 cup brown rice
- 4 oz skinless and boneless chicken fillet
- 1/2 tbsp coconut oil
- 1/2 cup cashew nuts
- 2 shallot onions, chopped
- 3.5 oz green beans
- 1/2 yellow bell pepper, sliced finely
- 1/2 red bell pepper, sliced finely
- 1/2 cup oyster mushrooms
- 2 tbsp lime juice
- 1 tbsp tahini
- 1/4 inch fresh ginger root, finely grated

## Directions:

Boil the rice with a cup of water and then simmer on a medium heat until it is fluffy and cooked. Lightly toast the cashews nuts in a dry pan. Heat a frying pan with the coconut oil over a medium heat, add the onions and cook until they are browning. Then place the chicken in the pan to stir-fry it. Stir in the green beans, bell peppers and mushrooms until they start to soften. Thoroughly mix together the lime juice, tahini and ginger root.

Add this paste to the chicken and vegetables, toss with the cashew nuts. Serve the chicken over a bed of brown rice.

# Thursday: Breakfast

<u>Porridge with chia seed, raisins and goji berries</u>

## Ingredients:

- 2 cups oats
- 3 cups almond milk
- 1 tbsp chia seeds
- 1 tbsp raisins
- 1 tbsp goji berries
- 2 tsp agave syrup

## Directions:

Place the oats and milk in a saucepan and bring to the boil, before turning it to a medium heat. Add in the chia seed, raisins and goji berries. Continue to stir the porridge until it is soft and cooked. Add more milk if the porridge becomes too dry. Serve in a large, flat bowl and top with a whirl of agave syrup to taste.

# Thursday: Lunch

<u>Pumpkin and squash soup</u>

## Ingredients:

- 6oz butternut squash, halved, deseeded
- 6oz pumpkin, halved, deseeded
- Canola oil
- 1/2 tbsp coconut oil
- 1 tbsp canola oil
- 1 small red onion, thinly sliced
- 200ml chicken stock
- 40ml coconut milk
- 40ml 2% milk
- 1/2 tsp parsley
- 1/2 tsp coriander

## Directions:

Heat the oven to 200 degrees celsius. Garnish the squash and pumpkin with canola oil and bake in the oven for at least 90 minutes until really soft. Let the vegetables cool down. Scoop out the squash and the pumpkin. Heat the coconut oil with the canola on medium heat and add the red onion, fry until golden. In a blender, puree together the pumpkin, squash, onions and half of the stock. Move this puree to another large pot and add the remaining stock. Simmer the mixture. Add the coconut milk, 2% milk, coriander and parsley.

# Thursday: Dinner

<u>Green tofu curry with sweet potatoes</u>

## Ingredients:

- 1 can coconut milk (light)
- 4 oz sweet potato, cubed
- 1/2 tbsp fish sauce
- 1 tsp himalayan salt
- 3 cloves garlic, crushed
- 1 tbsp canola oil
- 1 tbsp green curry paste
- 1/2 packet extra-firm tofu, sliced into 1/2 inch cubes
- 1/2 red bell pepper
- 1 cup frozen peas
- 2 tbsp lime juice
- Small handful coriander, roughly chopped.
- 2 scallions spring onions

## Directions:

Boil the sweet potatoes until they are ever so slightly soft. Heat the canola oil in a large saucepan on a medium to high heat and add the garlic, curry paste and tofu. Fry well until golden brown all over. Drop the heat slightly and add the peppers and peas. Wait until the peppers are slightly softened, then add the potatoes, coconut milk, fish sauce and salt. Stir this mixture well but gently. Add the lime juice and spring onions before serving and garnish with some coriander.

# Friday: Breakfast

<u>Fruit salad with yoghurt</u>

## Ingredients:

- 1 kiwi
- 1 apricot
- Handful red grapes
- 1/2 papaya
- 1/2 green apple
- 1/4 cup fresh coconut, grated
- 1 cup low fat natural yoghurt

## Directions:

Dice the kiwi, apricot and papaya into small cubes. Halve the grapes and finely slice the apple. Mix all the fruit together with the yoghurt, sprinkle with the grated coconut.

# Friday: Lunch

<u>Tempeh with lentils and greens</u>

## Ingredients:

- 3/4 cup lentils
- 4oz tempeh (1/2 pack), finely sliced
- 1 tbsp olive oil
- 2 scallions shallots
- 1/2 cup mustard greens, finely chopped
- 1 cup asparagus, chopped
- 3 radishes, halved and finely sliced
- 1 cup spinach leaves, chopped
- 1 cup rocket leaves, chopped

*Dressing*

- 1 tbsp olive oil
- 1 tbsp lemon juice
- 1 tsp agave

## Directions:

Boil the lentils until soft. Drain and cool. Turn a saucepan to medium-high heat and add the olive oil. Fry the tempeh on both sides until golden brown and slightly crisping. Allow to cool. Fry the shallots until cooked, then put to the side. Steam the asparagus until slightly cooked. Mix together the tempeh, lentils, shallots, asparagus, radishes and all the other greens. Stir together the olive oil, lemon juice and agave. Dress the salad.

# Friday: Dinner

<u>Satay chicken with wild rice and tomato salad</u>

## Ingredients:

- 4oz boneless, skinless chicken fillet, cubed
- 1/2 cup wild rice
- 1/2 cup cherry tomatoes, halved
- 1tbsp basil leaves, chopped

*Satay sauce:*

- 1/2 cup roasted peanuts
- 1/4 cup water
- 1 small garlic clove, crushed
- 1 tsp himalayan salt
- 1 tsp olive oil
- 1 tsp sesame seeds
- 1 tbsp agave syrup
- 1 tbsp fish sauce
- 1 tsp lime juice
- 1 pinch paprika
- 1/4 cup coconut milk

## Directions:

Bring the rice to the boil and then simmer until it is fluffy and cooked. To make the sauce, blend all the satay ingredients in a blender until they run smooth. Marinate the chicken in the satay sauce for 15 minutes. Place the chicken on two skewers and cook them in a pan on a medium-hot heat. Add the rest of the sauce if there is any left over. Garnish the tomatoes with some basil leaves and place on the plate with the rice and chicken skewers

# Saturday: Breakfast

Power smoothie and raw muesli

## Ingredients:

*Muesli*:

- 1/4 cup oats
- 1/4 cup spelt flakes
- 1/4 cup rye flakes
- 1/4 cup pre-cooked wheat berries
- 1 tbsp cranberries
- 1 tbsp raisins
- 1 tbsp roasted pumpkin seeds

*Smoothie:*

- 6 inches fresh root ginger
- 5 carrots
- 4 inches turmeric

## Directions:

To make the muesli, mix together all the muesli ingredients. Pour over milk of your choice. To make the smoothie, place all the smoothie ingredients through a juicer. Pour the ingredients into a glass. Add a straw and a cube of ice and feel re-energised!

# Saturday: Lunch

<u>Mushroom and spinach omelette</u>

## Ingredients:

- 4 eggs
- 1 tsp himalayan salt
- 1 tbsp olive oil
- 2 handfuls baby spinach leaves
- 1 cup brown mushrooms chopped

## Directions:

Turn the pan to medium-heat with the olive oil.
Add the spinach and mushrooms and fry until fully
softened. Spread the contents of the pan evenly
with some room around the edge. In the meantime,
crack four eggs into a bowl and whisk fully. Add
salt to the mixture. Pour the egg mixture into the
saucepan on high heat. Allow the egg to cook and
use a spatula to 'pick up' the egg around the sides
as it hardens. Without breaking the egg, fold the
omelette circle over to create a 'semi-circle'. Ensure
the egg is cooked fully, and to your liking before
serving. Serve with toast, spread with coconut
butter.

# Saturday: Dinner

## Tuna salad with orange and pomegranate

**Ingredients:**

- 4 oz tuna fillet, in chunks
- 2 tsp himalayan salt
- 1 tbsp agave syrup
- 1 tsp paprika
- 1 clove garlic, crushed
- 1 inch garlic root, finely chopped
- 1 red bell pepper
- 1 cup red chard, finely chopped
- 1/2 cup romaine lettuce finely chopped
- 1 tbsp olive oil
- 1 tbsp pomegranate seeds
- 1/2 orange, zested and juiced

**Directions:**

Mix the salt, agave, paprika, garlic and ginger together with the orange juice and zest. Soak the tuna in the mixture for about 10 minutes to marinade. Mix up the red chard and bell pepper into a bowl. Fry the marinated tuna until fully cooked through. Then, add the red chard and pepper; fry for a few more minutes. Place the cooked stir fry on top of the lettuce and sprinkle with olive oil and pomegranate seeds.

# Sunday: Breakfast

A cup of green tea and millet porridge with
flaxseed and plum topping.

## Ingredients:

- 2 cups millet flakes
- 3 cups 2% milk
- 2 tbsp flaxseed
- 2 plums, destoned
- 1 tbsp agave syrup

## Directions:

Bring the millet flakes and flaxseed with milk to the
boil and then simmer on a low heat until fully
cooked. Puree the plums and the agave syrup
thoroughly in a blender. Serve the porridge in a
wide, shallow bowl and allow to cool slightly. Place
a dollop of plum puree on top in the centre.

# Sunday: Lunch

<u>Chicken, beetroot and kale salad</u>

## Ingredients:

- 4 oz boneless, skinless chicken fillet, cubed
- 1/2 cup broccoli chopped
- 1/2 cup beetroot grated
- 1 avocado
- 1 handful kale chopped
- himalayan sea salt
- 1 tbsp roasted sunflower seeds
- 1 tbsp lemon juice
- 1 tsp paprika

## Directions:

Fry the chicken cubes in olive oil and allow to cool.
Steam the broccoli spears until slightly soft.
Massage the kale throughly with the avocado and
salt. Add the chicken, broccoli, beetroot and kale
with avocado. Top with sunflower seeds. Mix up
the lemon juice and paprika and pour over the
salad to dress.

# Sunday: Dinner

<u>Sardines with mint and greens</u>

## Ingredients:

- 1 tsp paprika
- 1 inch fresh ginger root
- 2 tbsp tahini paste
- 2 tbsp agave syrup
- 6 sardines, heads removed
- 1 small handful coriander, chopped
- 2 scallions spring onion
- 1/2 cup collard greens, chopped
- 1/2 cup baby spinach
- 1/2 cup chopped mint

## Directions:

Mix the tahini, paprika, ginger, mint and agave. Cut across the skin of the fish on each side and place in a shallow dish. Poor the tahini sauce all over the fish. Broil the dish for 10 minutes until it is fully cooked. In the meantime, lightly fry the spring onion, and steam the collard greens and spinach. Serve the sardines garnished with the spring onion and coriander next to the steamed vegetables.

# CONCLUSION

As our bodies and minds are increasingly forced to face a barrage of pollutants and chemicals as a result of living in modern society, it is important that we take our physical and mental health into our own hands by seeking out the foods that help us to combat the cell damage caused by excessive free radicals.

Foods high in vitamins, minerals and antioxidants-superfoods-are our best defense. When you fill your diet with foods that are nutrient-rich, filling and healthy, there is less room for the high-sugar, processed foods that, instead of contributing to the vitality and health of your body and mind, only strip it away, leaving you lethargic and fuzzy.

Excellent brain health, mental vitality, not to mention an improved mood is what you have to look forward to. Now that you've completed the guide, found your favorite superfoods and made of a list of a few you want to try, choose the recipes you would like to experiment with this week and make your grocery list.

In order to get the most out of the foods you've read about in this guide, seek out reputable sources of food, buying organic produce, oils and grains, and opting for responsibly farmed meats, as well as fish that is wild caught. As you shop, stick to the perimeter of the store where the freshest foods are located.

By learning about the health-enhancing properties of each of the superfoods contained in this guide, you equip yourself to make the best possible choices about what kinds of foods you put in your mouth in order to fuel your body and your mind. In doing this you do your part to take charge of your health goals and to feel the best you ever have. A superfood diet takes you there.

# LIKE THIS REPORT?

Thanks for downloading and reading this report. I'm positive if you just follow this plan, you will reach your health goals a lot easier and quicker than you realize. However, could you spare one minute and do me a quick favour though?

If you found this report useful, would you leave me a positive review on Amazon?

I love getting feedback and knowing I'm helping people makes a real difference to me. I read all my reviews and would really appreciate your thoughts. A 5 star review on Amazon is like giving me a tip for $20.

... And I would very, very much appreciate the gesture.

To leave a review, please visit:
http://bit.ly/superbrainfoods

Thanks again and I wish you the best of luck.

Your trusted friend,
Jennifer James